VIRAL VOCABULARY

An Illustrated Look at the Language of the COVID-19 Pandemic

EMILY POGERS
MAUREEN CASAMASSIMO

2021 First Paperback Edition

Copyright © 2021 by Emily Pogers and Maureen Casamassimo

Illustrations © 2021 by Paul Casamassimo

All rights reserved. The text and/or illustrations may not be reproduced without written permission of copyright holders.

This book is presented solely for educational and entertainment purposes. The information is not intended as medical advice.

Quotes included in this book are attributed to the sources shown when doing an internet search on the specific topics discussed.

Library of Congress Control Number: 2021910168
ISBN 978-0-578-89746-2

Design by Dory Pogers

The text is set in Mrs. Eaves & Mr. Eaves

Published by E. Pogers, USA

DEDICATION

To our neighbors defeated by COVID-19,
most alone but some thankfully surrounded
by loved ones on FaceTime,

To the devoted medical workers who guided the
sick through the valley of COVID-19,

To the courageous hard-working people who
abruptly found themselves deemed essential,

To the leaders and media who preached
science and truth as the path forward, and

To the businesses that were shuttered peacefully
for the common good, as well as their workers,
left to wait for government help, fearing eviction,
and on ever-lengthening food lines.

THE YEAR 2029...

Henry and Thomas bounded off the school bus and into the house, excited because Pop and Mo should be in from Ohio. Thomas slammed the door and they ran up the stairs. Henry yelled "We're home," to what seemed to be an empty living room. Startled, Pop greeted them from the sofa where he had just nodded off over his tablet, "Hey guys, how was your day? Mo and Mom are shopping and I'm holding down the fort. Those backpacks look pretty heavy. Set them down and tell me what's cookin'."

Thomas said, "I'm hungry. I'll be right back."

Henry dropped his stuff and plopped down next to Pop. "Remember, I told you about my friend, Brie Loughlin. She's my Biology lab partner. She passed me a note in class today asking if I'd like to see *Godzilla and T-Rex* on Saturday. I'm so excited! Besides that, I ran the best mile in gym class! It was a pretty good day until my Language Arts and History teacher assigned a research paper. I have to choose an event in history that happened in my lifetime.

Would you be able to help me? I'd like to write about the Pandemic of 2020." Pop agreed, "Sure, we haven't worked together since we practiced the alphabet when you were little. Remember all those ABC books we read together?"

Thomas returned with the platter of Buckeye Treats. "Give us some," said Pop, "we can share the blame. Mo was saving them for dessert tonight." Thomas squished in next to the others like they used to when Pop read stories to them.

And then Pop began…

AT HOME

By mid-March 2020 many localities advised residents to shelter at home.

When possible, non-essential workers worked from home and students learned through online instruction.

Playgrounds, beaches, churches, parks, and border crossings were CLOSED.

Visitors were not allowed in hospitals and nursing homes.

"There is nothing like staying at home for real comfort."
– JANE AUSTEN

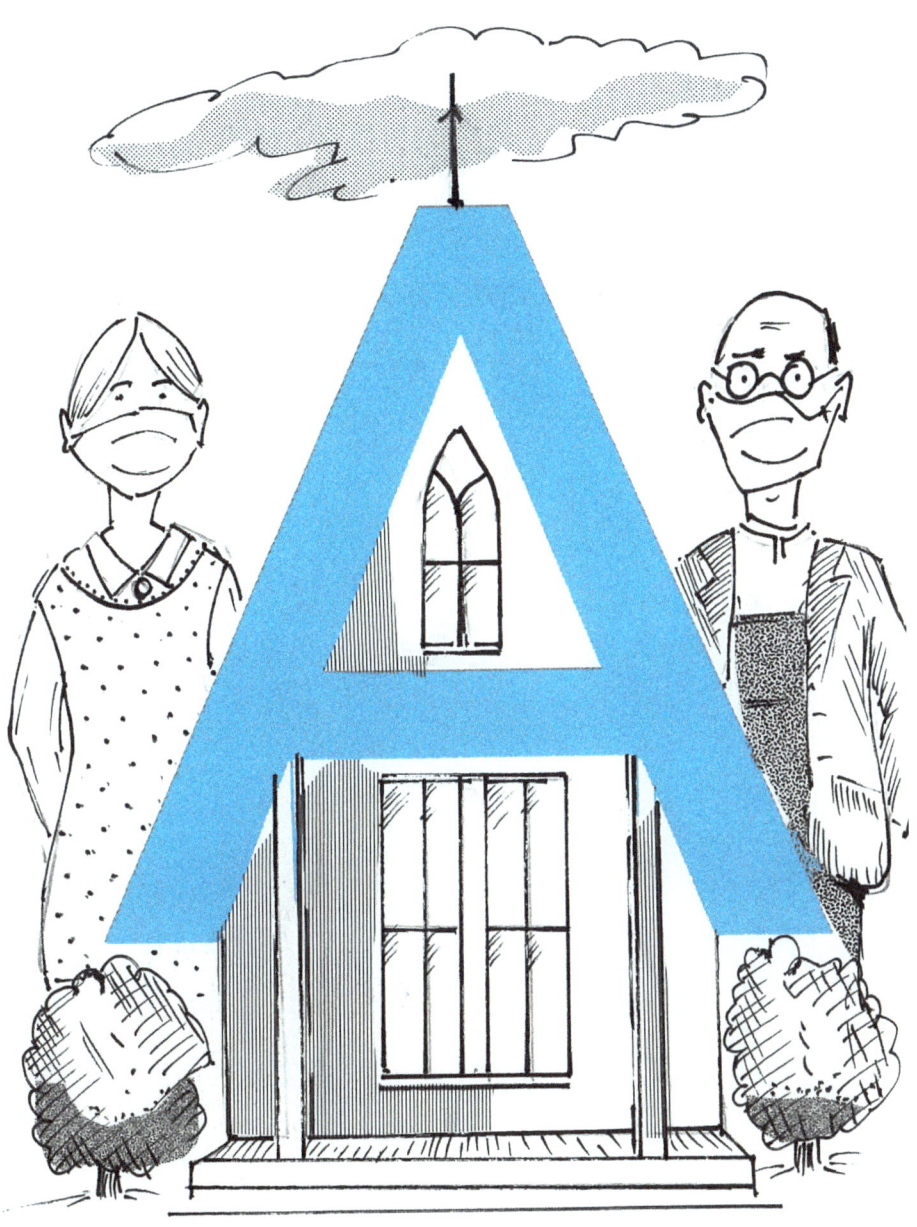

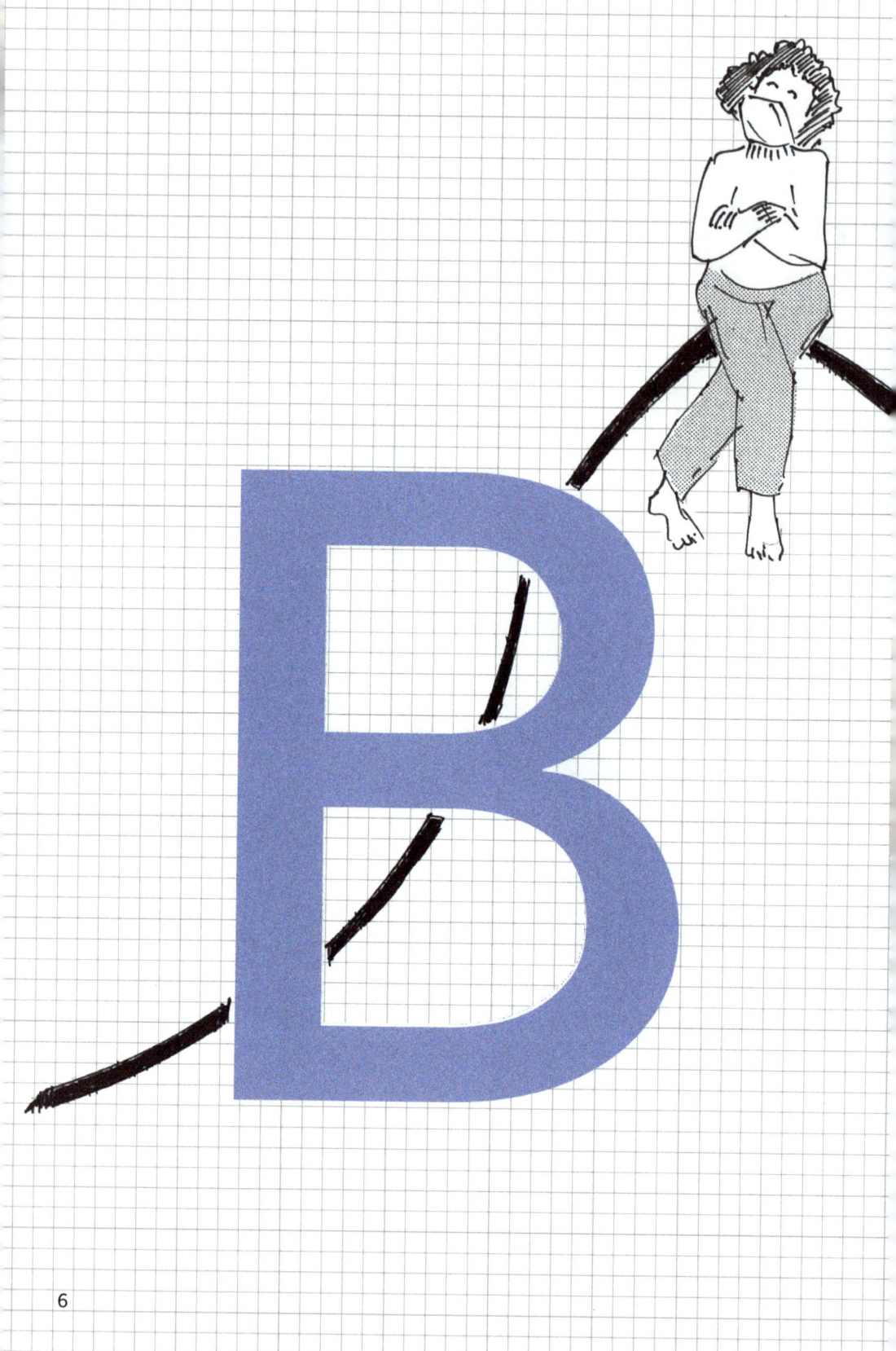

BENDING THE CURVE

The line graph of Disease Cases vs Time became less steep as more people took measures to stay at home, wash their hands and wear a mask in public.

Daily briefings by governors, mayors, and the President's task force referenced the progress in flattening and bending down the curve as a sign of progress against the disease.

"There is a magic in graphs. The profile of a curve reveals in a flash a whole situation — the life history of an epidemic, a panic, or an era of prosperity. The curve informs the mind, awakens the imagination, convinces."
– HENRY D. HUBBARD

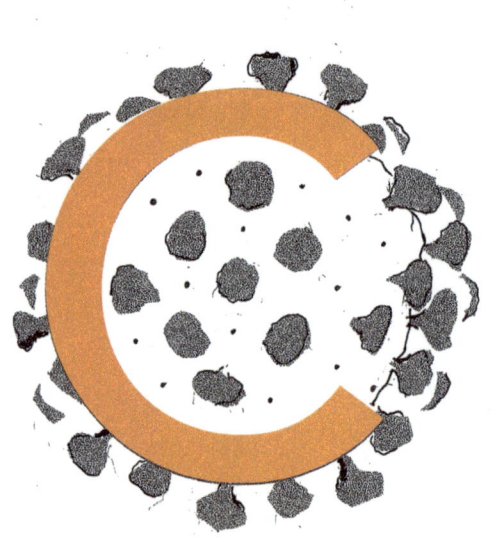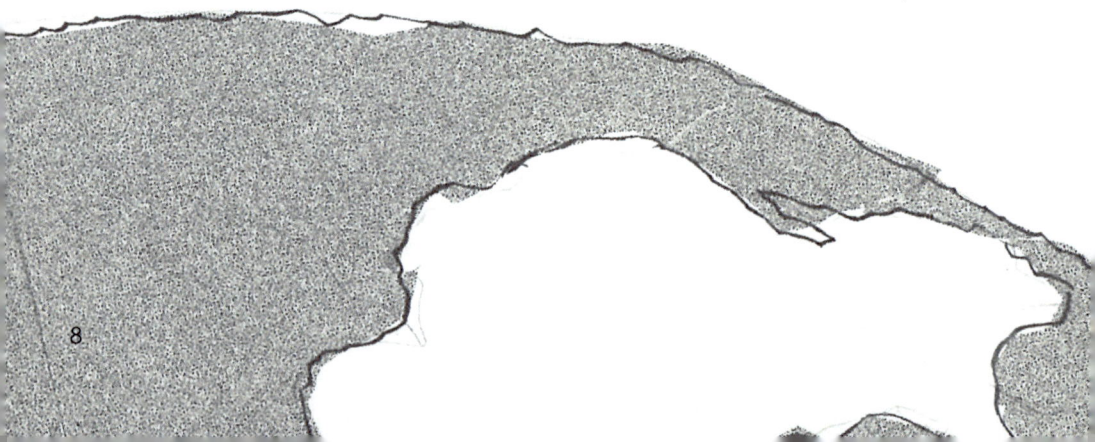

COVID-19

The cause of the worldwide outbreak of respiratory illness was a novel coronavirus.

It was known by the acronym for coronavirus disease of 2019, COVID-19.

The virus was believed to have started in Wuhan, China.

Conspiracy theorists claimed the pandemic was a hoax, but by midsummer 2020, almost 750,000 people worldwide had died.

"The worst potential bio-terrorist is nature itself."
– ANTHONY FAUCI

DISTANCING

Without treatments or a vaccine, health officials recommended keeping at least 6 feet apart.

Distancing was practiced throughout history to prevent the spread of disease, but the term "social distancing," was coined in 2020.

Businesses reduced capacity, enforced one-directional traffic flow, and applied floor stickers to help with distancing.

Restaurants built elaborate outdoor seating, hoping the increased capacity would enable them to stay open.

"There is nothing so strong or safe in an emergency of life as the simple truth." – CHARLES DICKENS

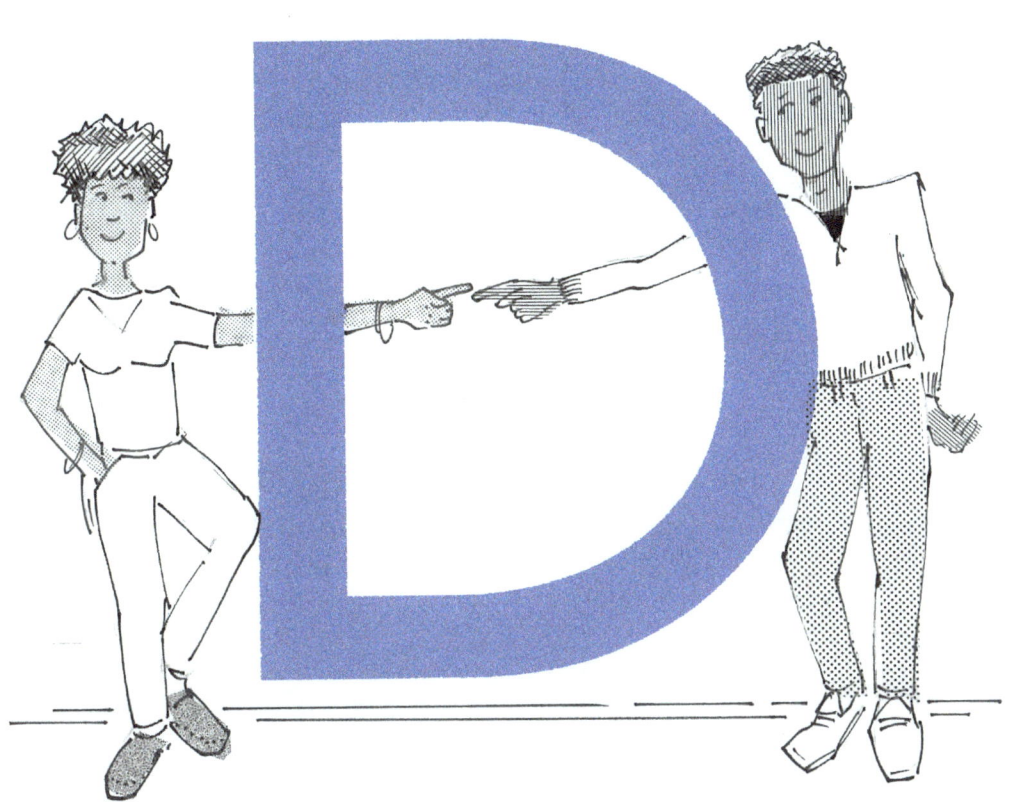

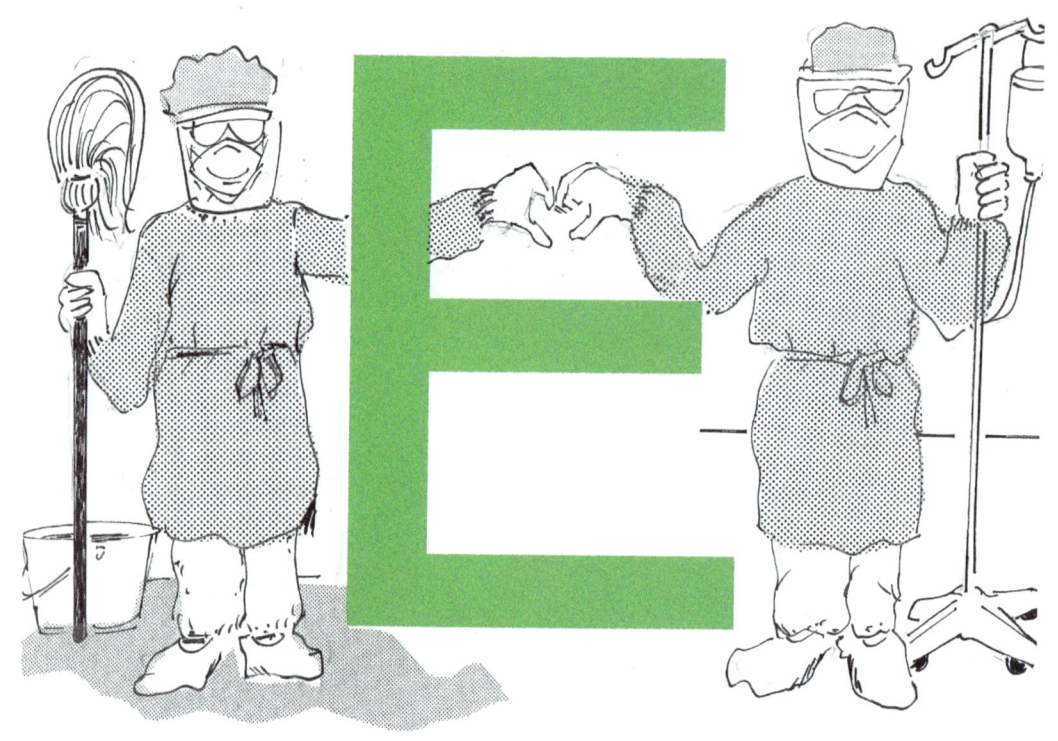

"Strength does not come from winning. Your struggles develop your strengths. When you go through hardships and decide not to surrender, that is strength."

– ARNOLD SCHWARZENEGGER

ESSENTIAL WORKERS

Governments labeled workers who conduct operations necessary to public health and safety as essential.

Essential workers cared for the sick, supplied our food, made deliveries, offered transportation, fought fires, cleaned shared spaces, and protected our communities.

Because working from home was not an option, daycare for the children of these families also became essential.

Many essential workers were on the front lines, and exposed themselves to COVID-19, yet they earned only the minimum wage.

FAUCI

Dr. Anthony Fauci, immunologist and a diminutive septuagenarian, was recognized and respected as one of the world's leading experts on infectious diseases.

He was considered by many to be America's "Mighty Mouse" on his way to save the day, as he led the war on the pandemic.

"I am a firm believer in the people... If given the truth, they can be depended upon to meet any national crisis. The great point is to bring them the real facts."
– ABRAHAM LINCOLN

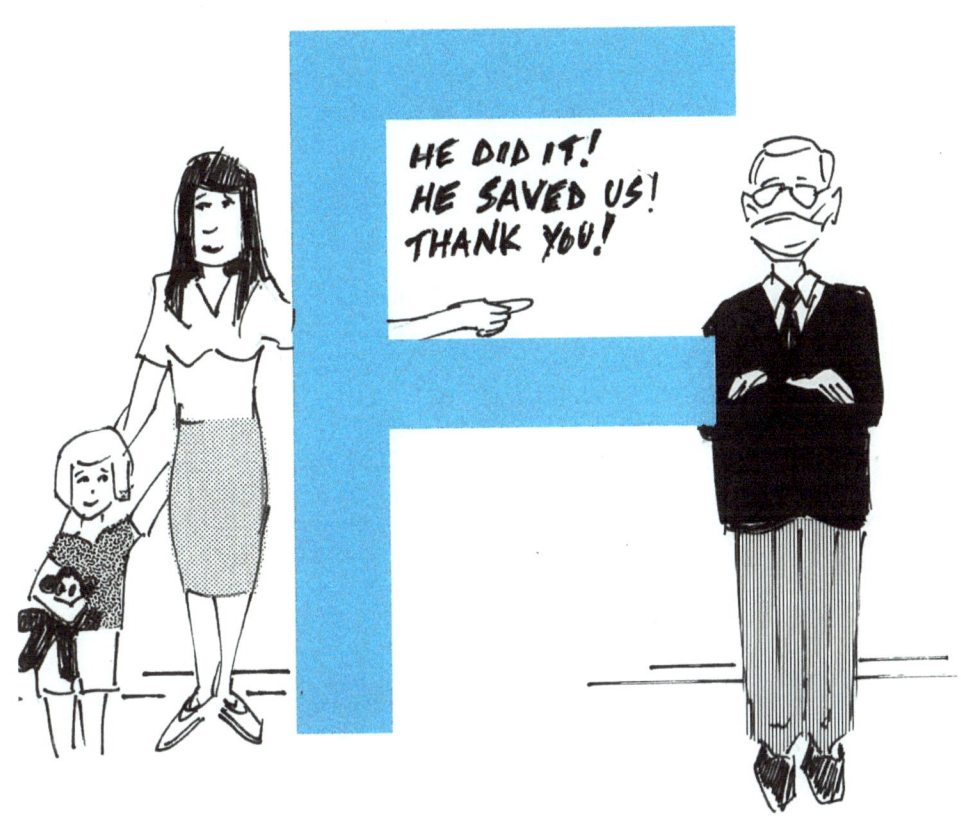

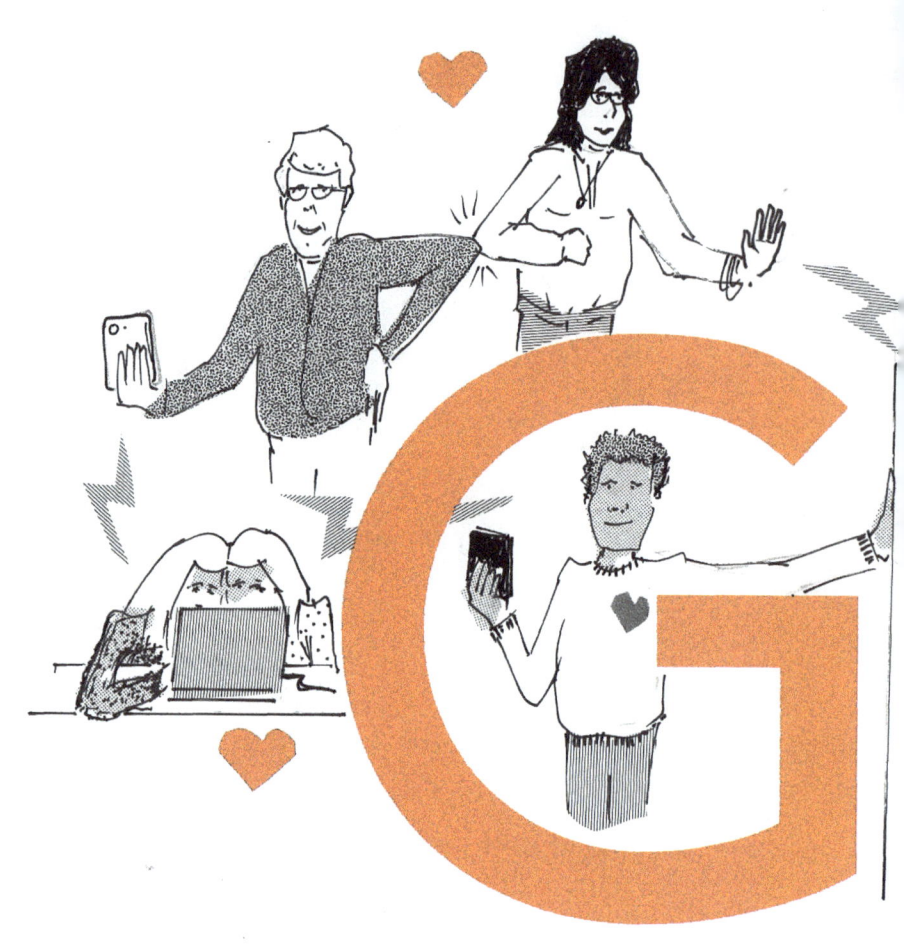

"Scatter Joy." – RALPH WALDO EMERSON

GREETINGS

Early on, elbow bumps replaced handshakes. Bumps were then replaced by waves, nods and shouts through masks.

Without in-person contact, feelings were expressed through emojis. Facial recognition with folks behind masks depended on eye contact.

Transactions were conducted through Plexiglass. Visits outside our "COVID pod" became more intimate, with hands on glass.

Birthday greetings were delivered by lawn signs, drive-by visits, and virtual parties.

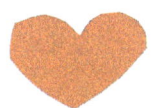

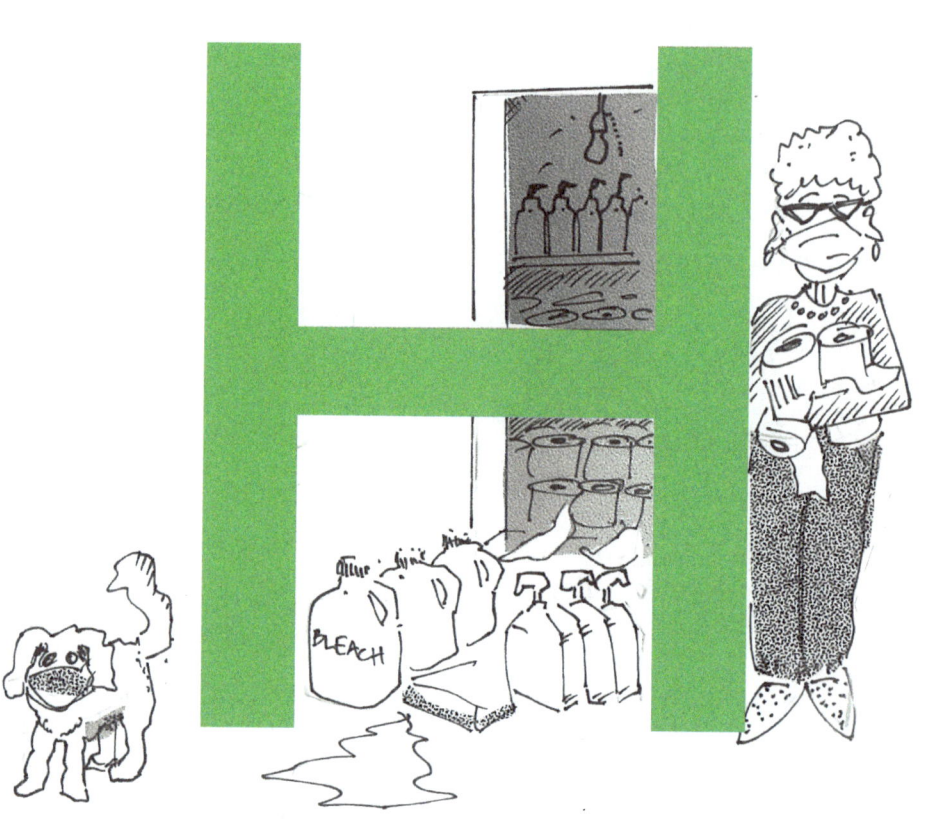

HOARDING

People felt a sense of urgency to stock up on supplies like toilet paper, masks and sanitizer.

Seeing others panic buy, they thought, "If they're doing it, I better do it too."

This led to scarcity and some people tried to make money by selling what they hoarded at inflated prices.

Businesses that increased prices to respond to demands were penalized.

"We are not cisterns made for hoarding, we are channels made for sharing." – BILLY GRAHAM

IMMUNITY

During the pandemic, it was unclear whether those who caught the virus could get it again, or acquire natural protection.

Transfusions of plasma from recovered COVID-19 patients seemed to help patients with active cases.

The world looked forward to herd immunity, when a large proportion of the population would be immune.

"Remember that time you got polio? No, you don't. Because your parents got you [bleep] vaccinated."
—JIMMY KIMMEL

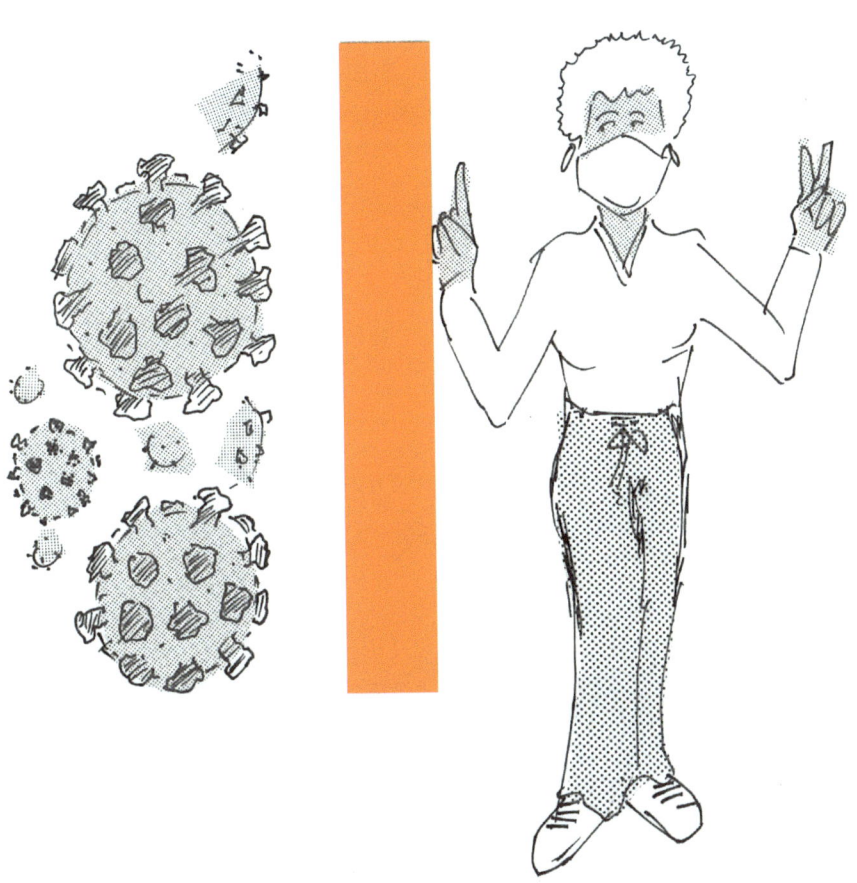

How do you describe Dr. Anthony at a COVID taskforce meeting?

Grouchi Fauci!

Did you see the COVID-19 joke on Twitter?

Yeah! It went viral...

Why is everyone faster after the pandemic?

Because we all Zoom!

JOKES

Humorous emails abounded to spread smiles during the stay at home order.

"Let us be grateful for the people who make us happy; they are the charming gardeners who make our souls blossom." – MARCEL PROUST

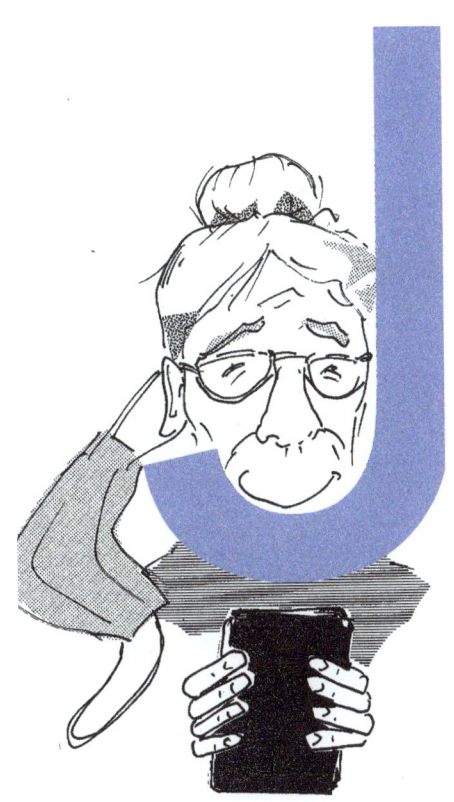

KINDNESS

In this stressful time some were moved to kindness. They looked out for neighbors, delivered goods, provided food and necessities.

Many continued in their jobs despite exposure to the virus because they wanted to help others. Wearing and making masks was a form of kindness and showed respect.

"Look for the helpers. You will always find people who are helping." – FRED ROGERS

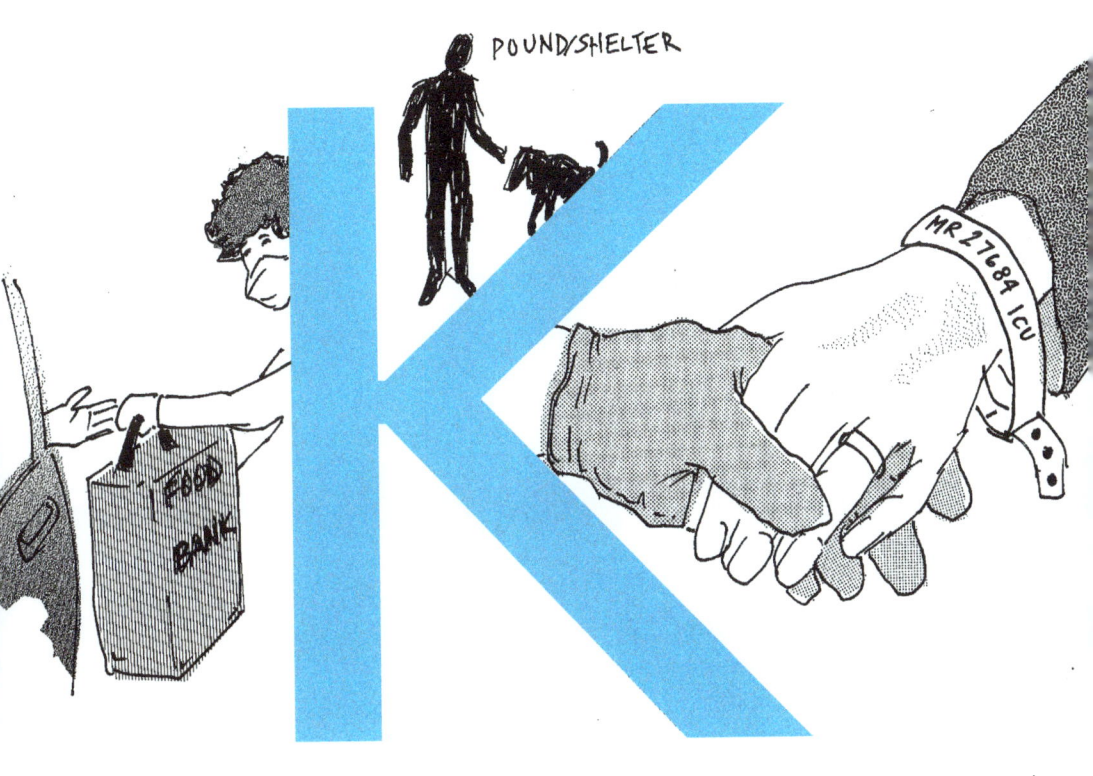

Patience is not simply the ability to wait - it's how we behave while we're waiting."

– JOYCE MEYER

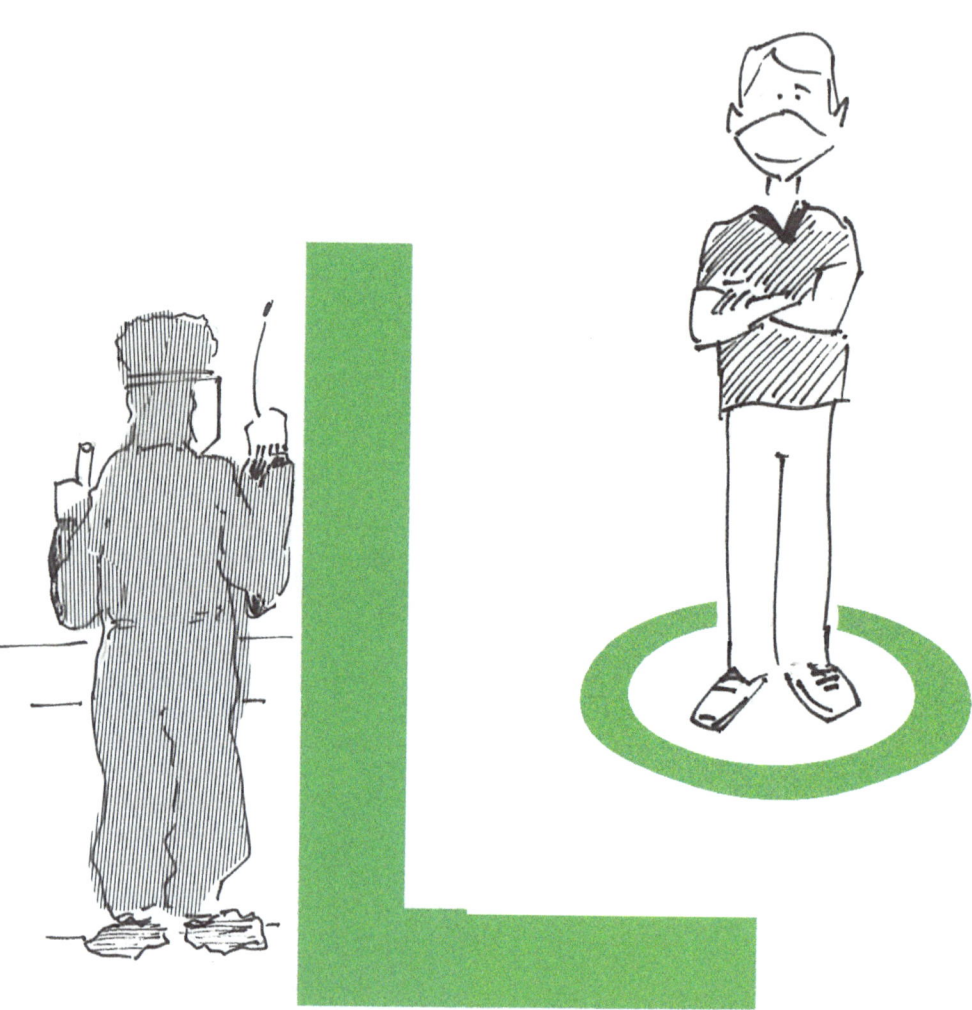

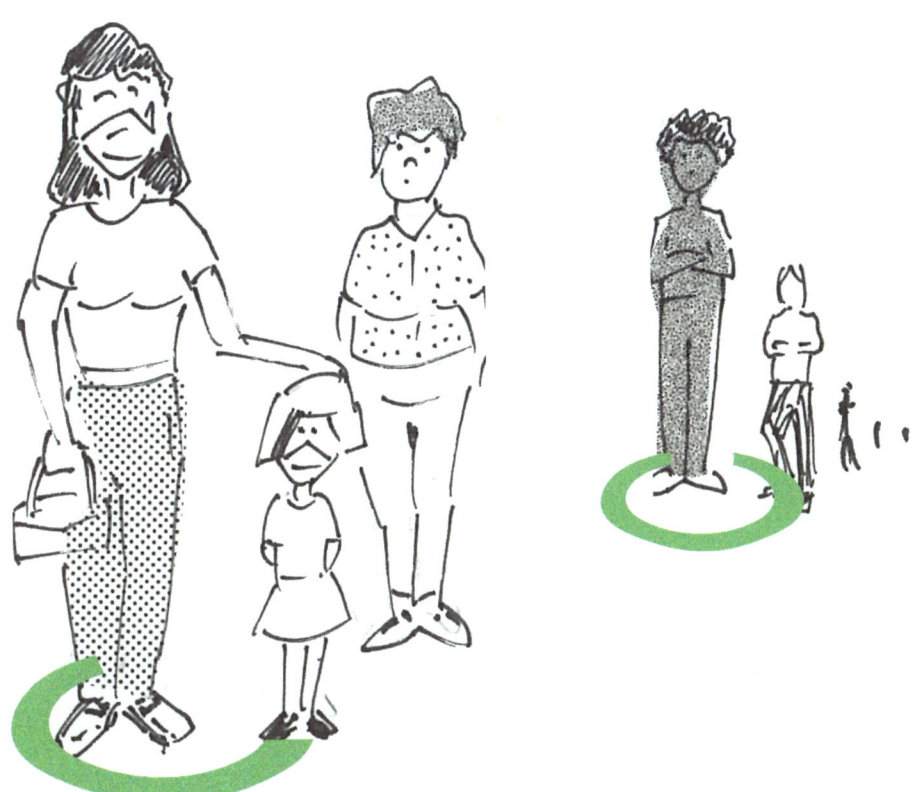

LINES

People and cars queued up for testing, grocery stores, food pantries, and vaccines while rows of coffins awaited burial at Potter's Field.

MASKS

These protections were a key component of personal protective equipment. First line workers used N95 masks that filtered at least 95% of particles at least 0.3 microns in size.

Face coverings for the general public were required or suggested in most areas. They became a fashion statement of the pandemic, an at-home crafting effort to contribute to the cause, and possibly an identification of your political "tribe."

"I wear a mask to protect you. You wear a mask to protect me." – DR. JAY C. BUTLER CDC

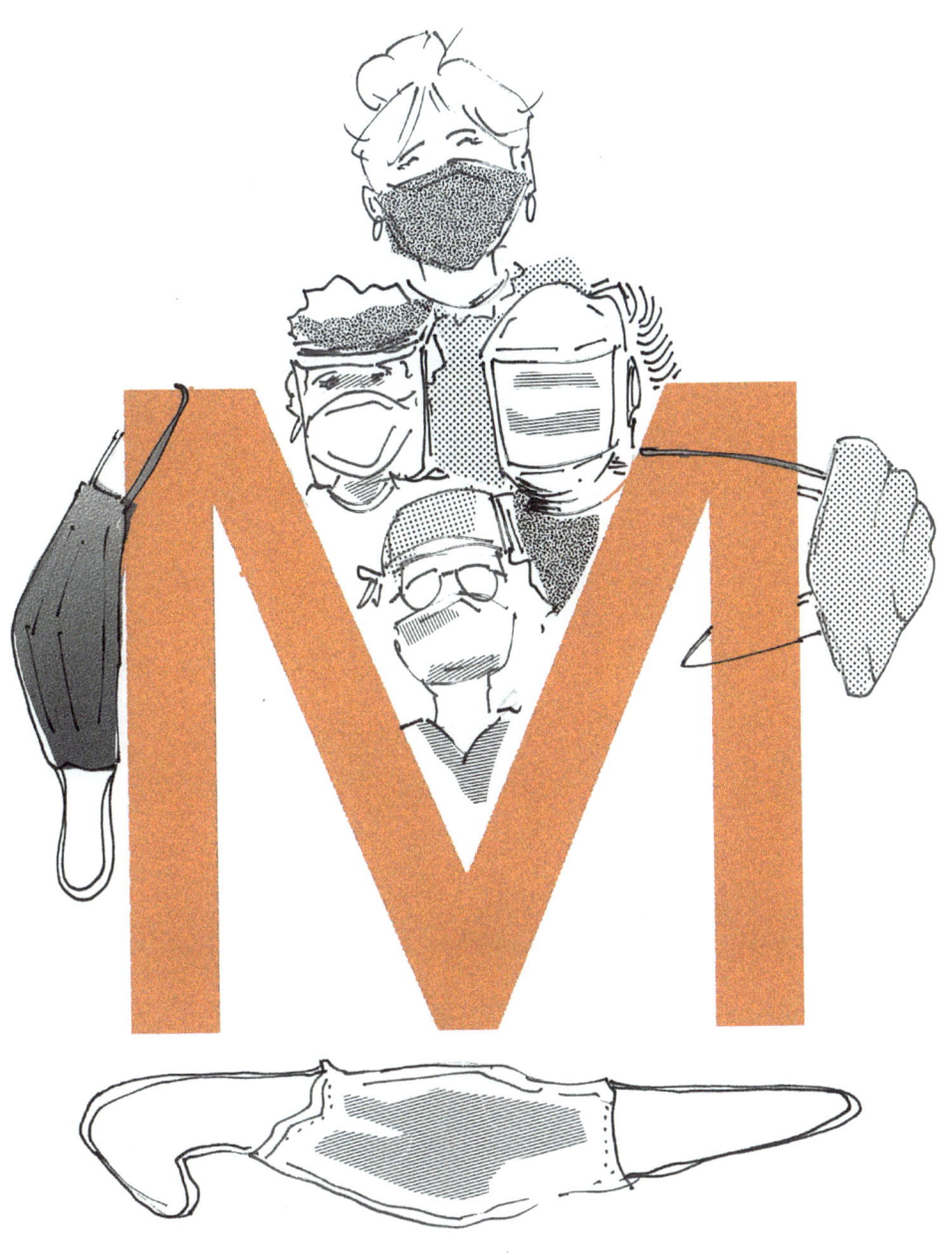

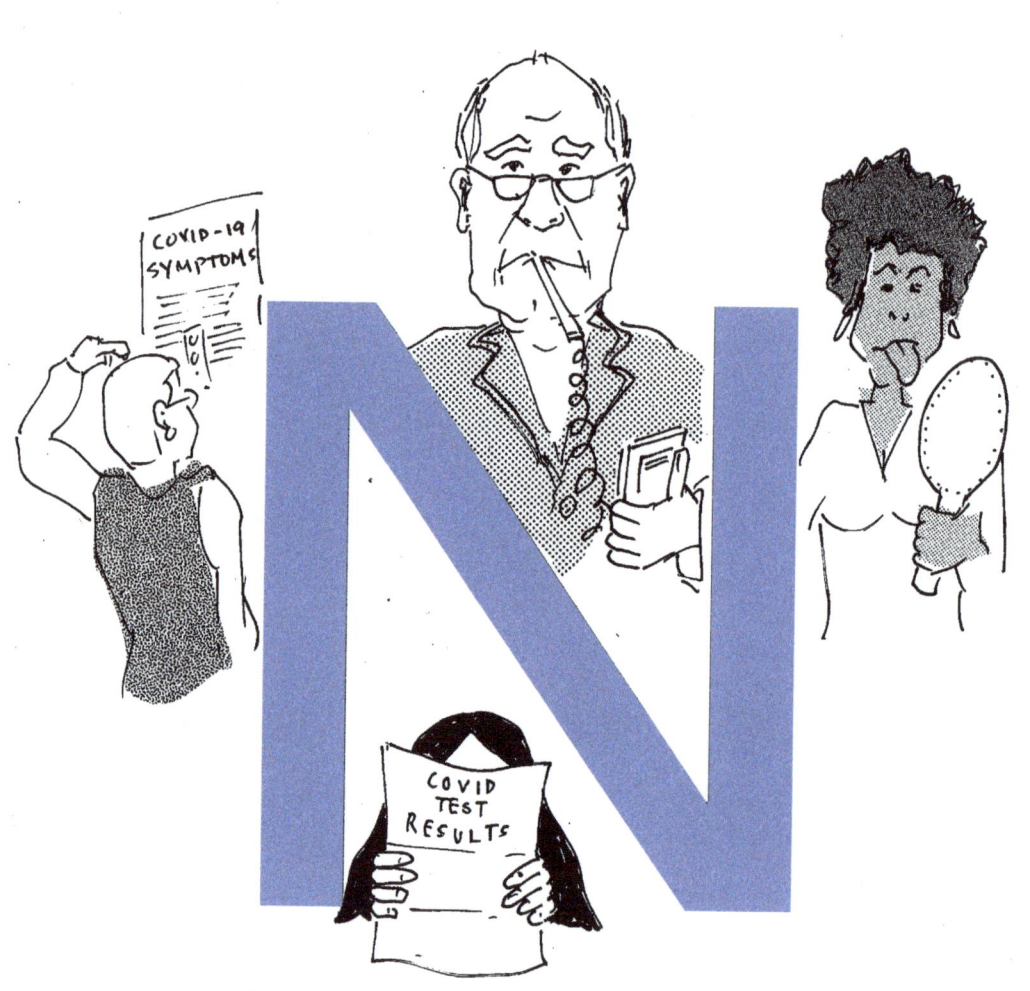

NON-SYMPTOMATIC

People without COVID-19 symptoms such as fever, cough, loss of taste and breathlessness still tested positive for the virus and could spread the disease to others.

"Appearances are often deceiving." – AESOP

OVERWHELMED

Communities worried that COVID-19 cases would overwhelm their healthcare systems.

As hospitals reached capacity, dedicated workers from elsewhere volunteered to help.

At home, individuals were challenged by the financial and emotional toll of the pandemic.

Morgues, funeral services and cemeteries were beyond stressed.

"Never give up, no matter how things look or how long they take. Don't quit before the miracle."
— ANNE LAMOTT nytimes.com

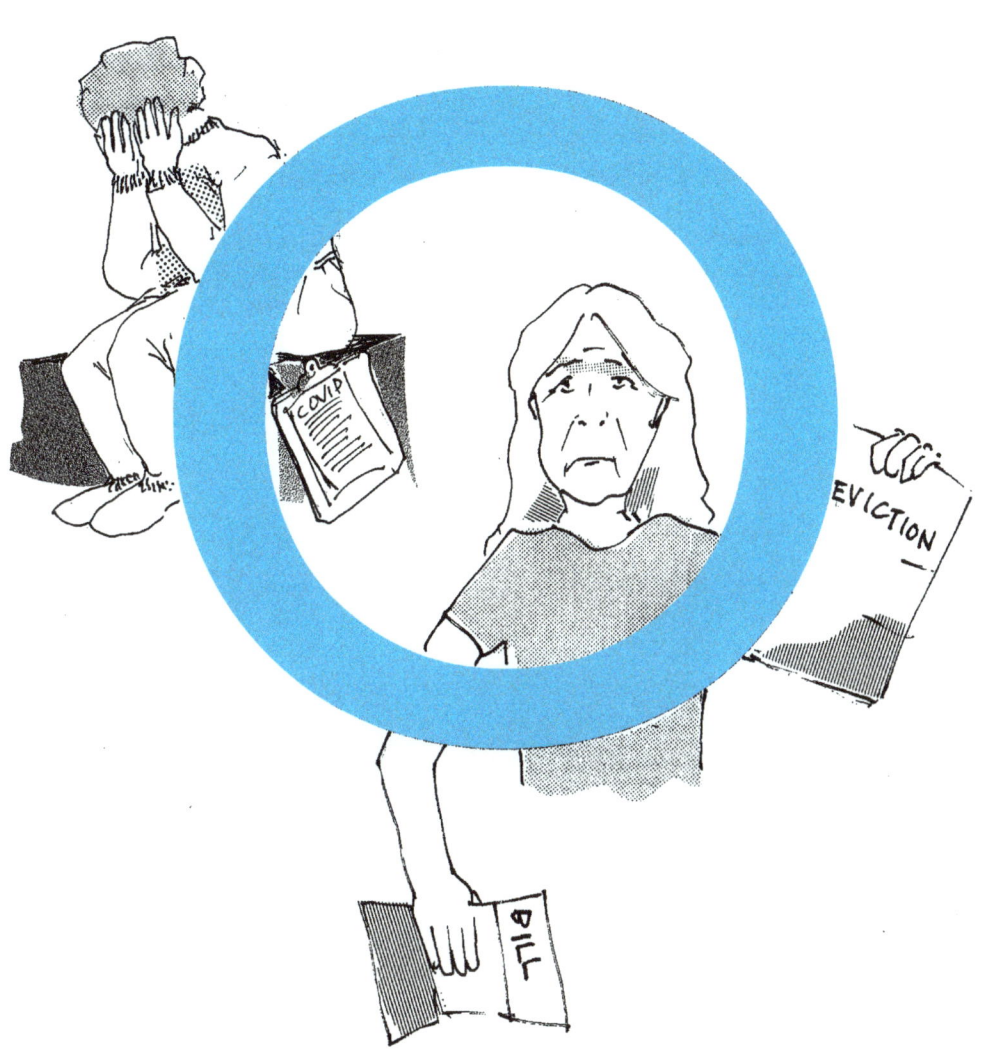

PREPAREDNESS

Despite warnings of an impending pandemic—the necessary plans, protective gear, testing supplies, hospital staffing and ventilators were not available.

Cities shut down abruptly, leaving businesses, schools and families to hastily develop strategies.

Some predicted the virus would come in waves which proved true.

"By failing to prepare, you are preparing to fail."
– BEN FRANKLIN

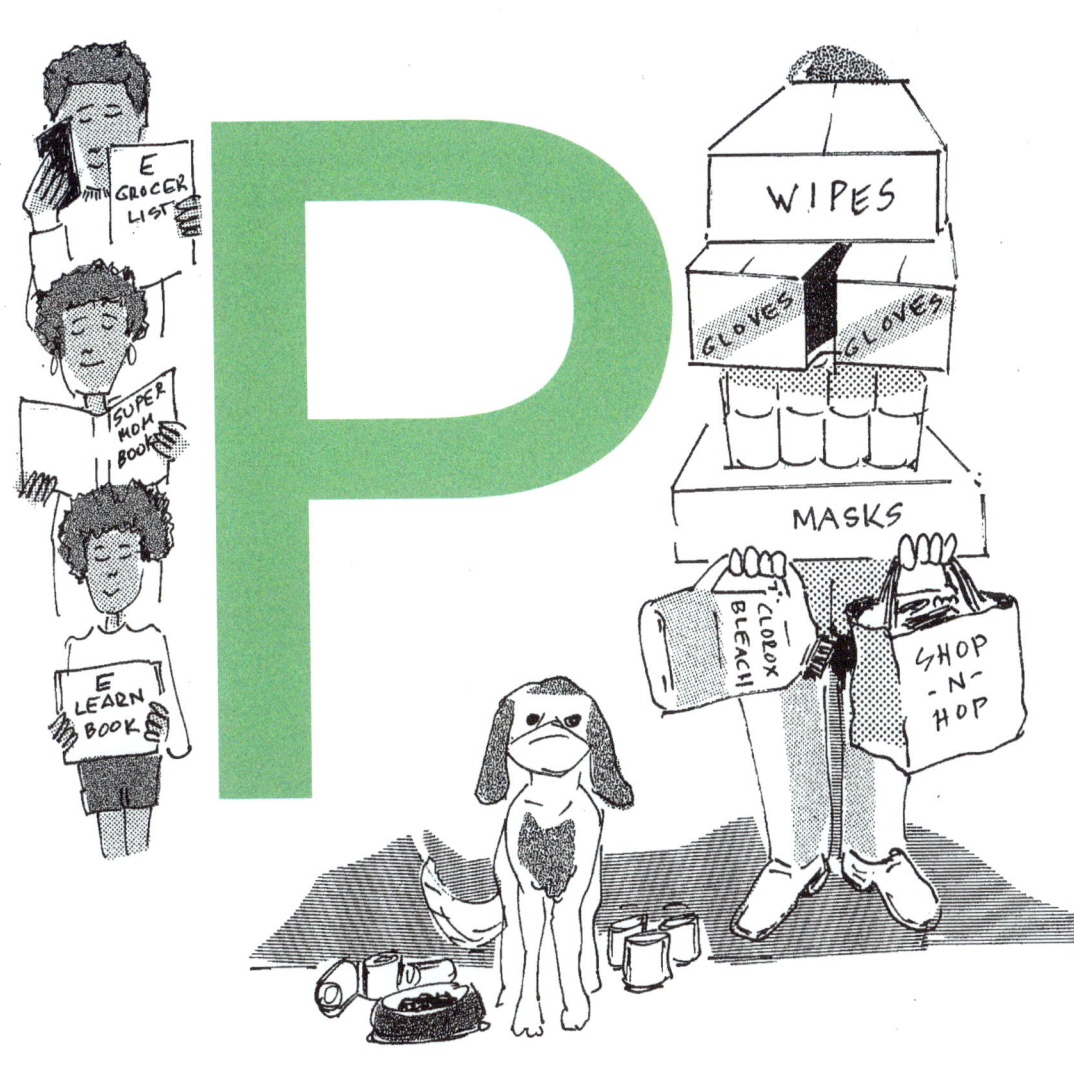

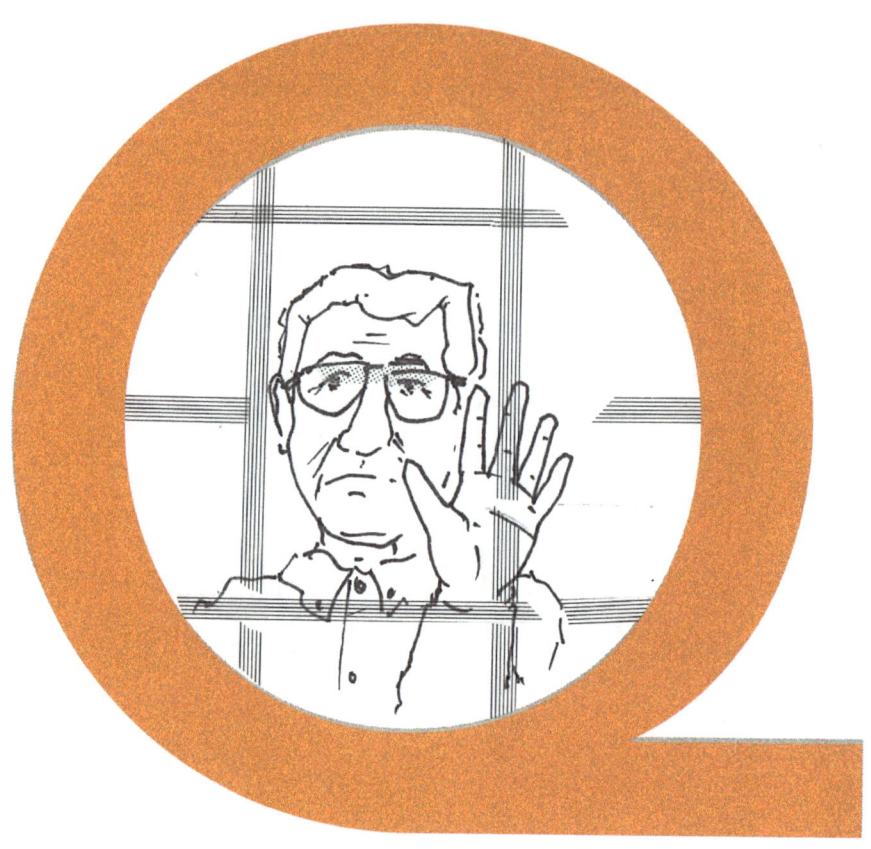

"My biggest worry is that, in the quiet before the storm, we forget how important every one of our choices is and how many lives we're impacting by what we are doing." – **DR. AMY ACTON**

ABC 6 Columbus, OH 04/02/2020

QUARANTINE

Quarantine, a centuries-old measure, meant isolating people believed to be infected.

People who were exposed to COVID-19 isolated on cruise ships, hotels, or in their own basements and bedrooms.

States with low incidence of infection required visitors from states with higher incidence to self-report and quarantine 14 days after arrival.

Some countries closed their borders to outsiders to control the spread.

REOPENING

Managing the correct balance between health and restoring the economy was contentious, as people wanted to get back to work and to socialize.

By fall of 2020, "COVID fatigue" was rampant and political denial regarding COVID-19, made unprotected mass gatherings frequent super-spreader events.

"Don't get cocky with COVID."
– ANDREW CUOMO

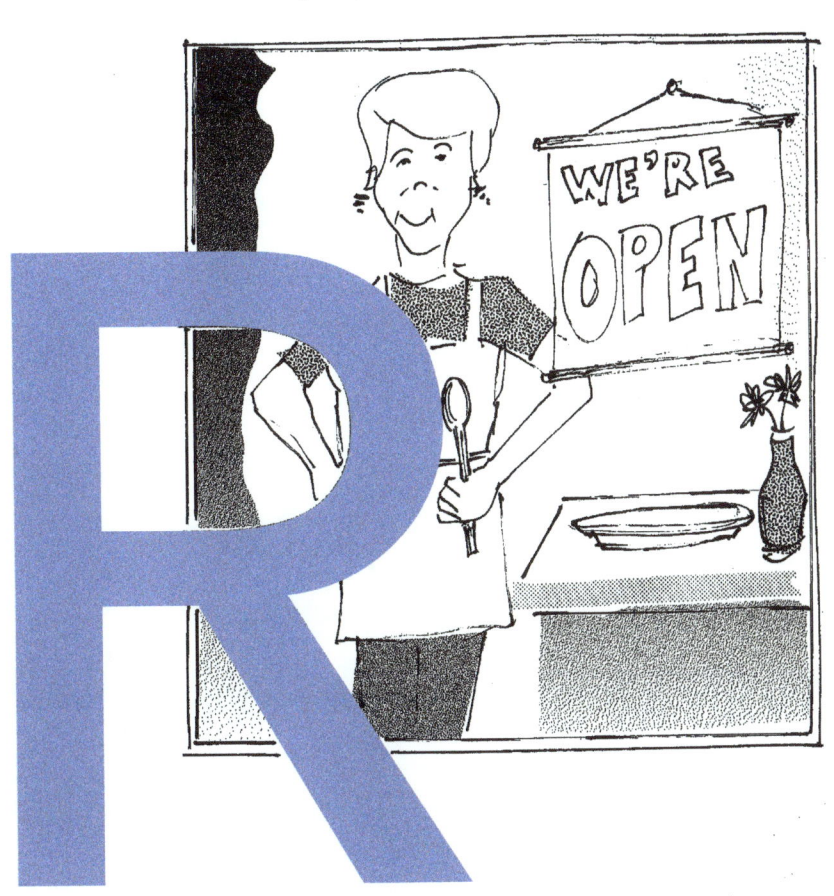

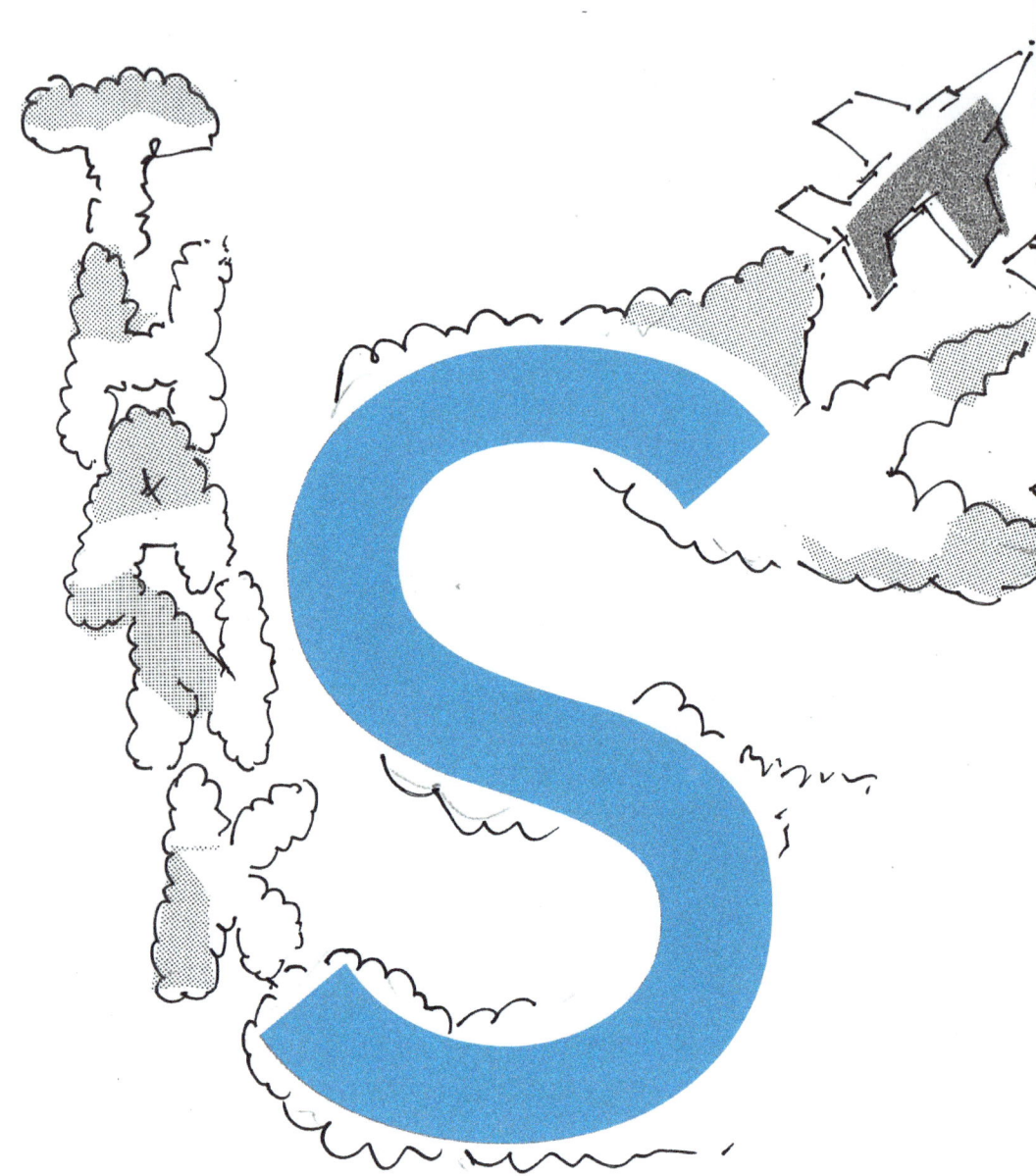

SALUTES

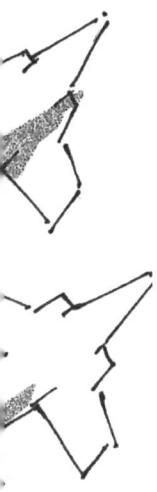

Communities, families, Blue Angels, Thunderbirds, and individuals expressed gratitude to frontline workers in organized flyovers, cheers, or music.

Each night at 7pm, it was time to salute the COVID-19 workers!

"Never doubt that a small group of thoughtful committed citizens can change the world. Indeed it is the only thing that ever has."

– MARGARET MEADE

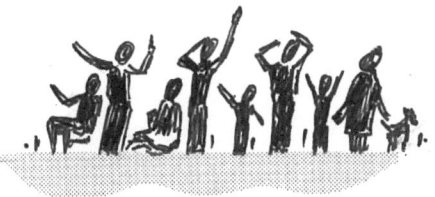

TESTING

Nasal swabs or saliva containing the virus were diagnostic of COVID-19 infection. Positive results required the individual to self-quarantine.

After recovery, people were tested to see if antibodies were in their blood.

Availability, accuracy and delays in obtaining results were all problematic throughout the pandemic. This prevented accurate contact tracing.

"All through my life I have been tested. My will has been tested, my courage has been tested, my strength has been tested. Now my patience and endurance are being tested." – MUHAMMAD ALI

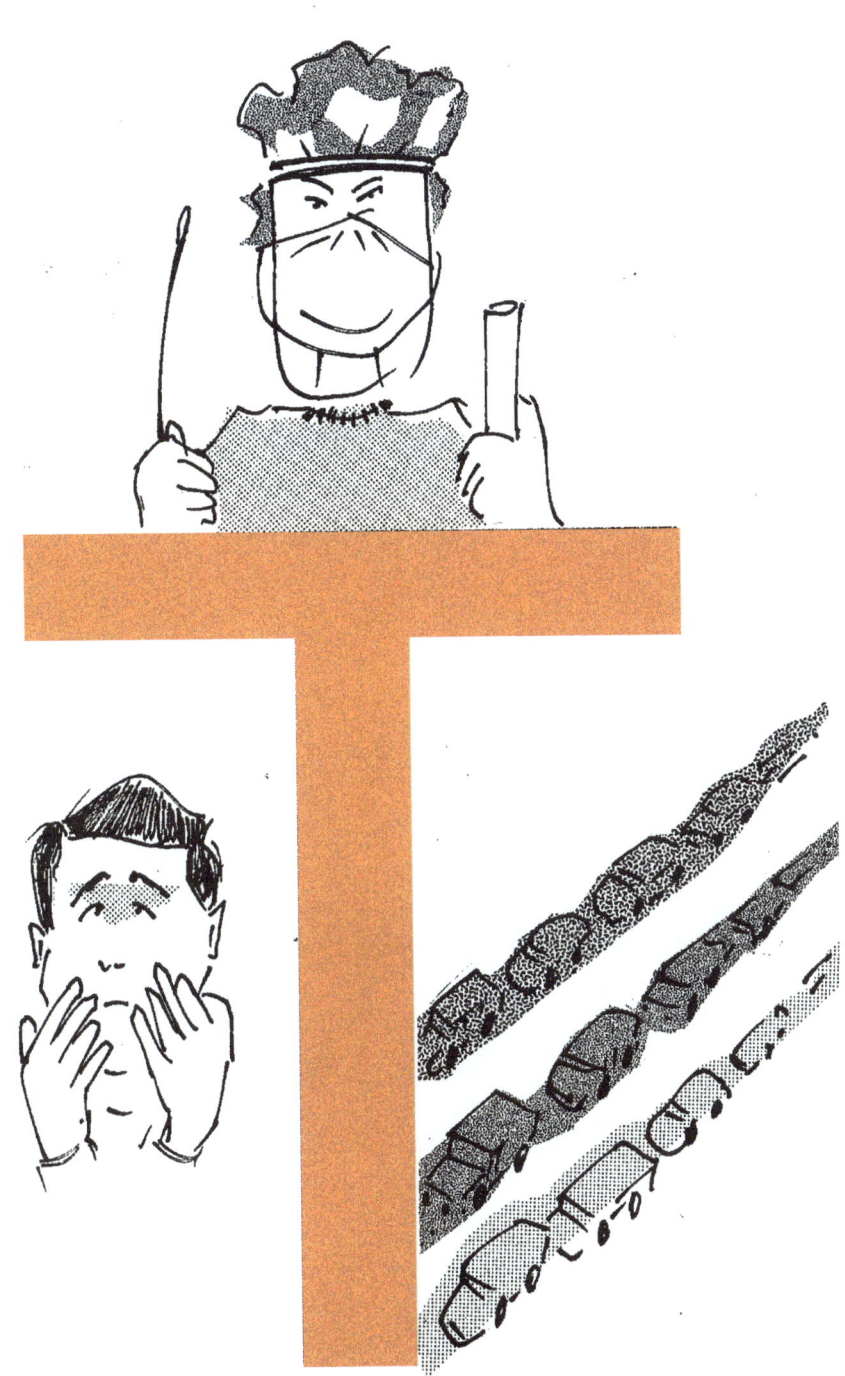

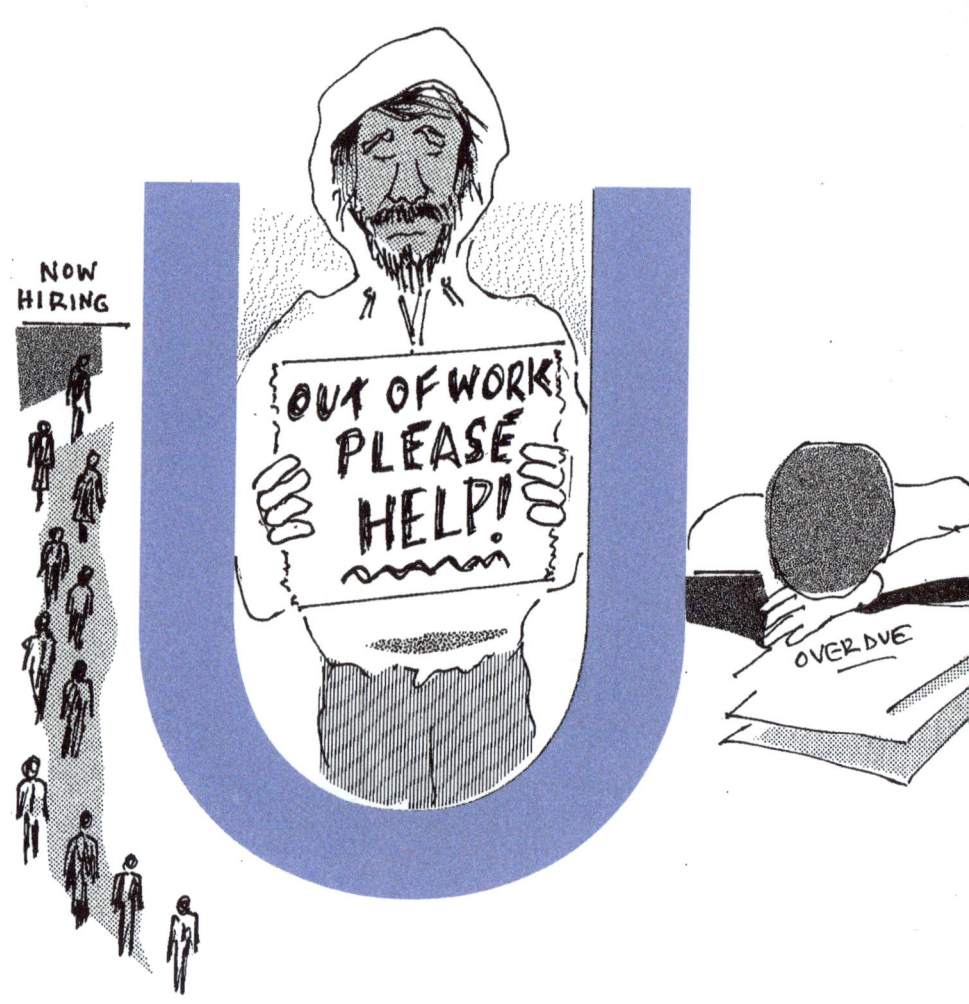

UNEMPLOYMENT

In April 2020, the out-of-work rate surged to 14.7%, the highest recorded since 1948. The rate was estimated to have been about 25% at the peak of the Great Depression in 1933.

State computer systems were overwhelmed by the number of people out of work and signing up for unemployment benefits.

Many businesses were forced to shut down for good. Given limitations on capacity, it proved impossible to make a profit.

"Life for many people, begins to crumble on the edges; but it is not, for all that, that we need abandon." – DOROTHEA LANGE

VENTILATOR

Patients with severe COVID-19 were put on ventilators to breathe.

The machines pumped oxygen through a tube, into the patients' mouths, down their windpipes, and into their lungs.

The tube was uncomfortable; while it was hooked up, one couldn't eat or talk. Nutrients were delivered through an IV.

An early worry was that the supply of ventilators would not be sufficient for all the suffering patients. Some hospitals adapted one machine to serve 2 patients.

Many people on a ventilator did not recover and died.

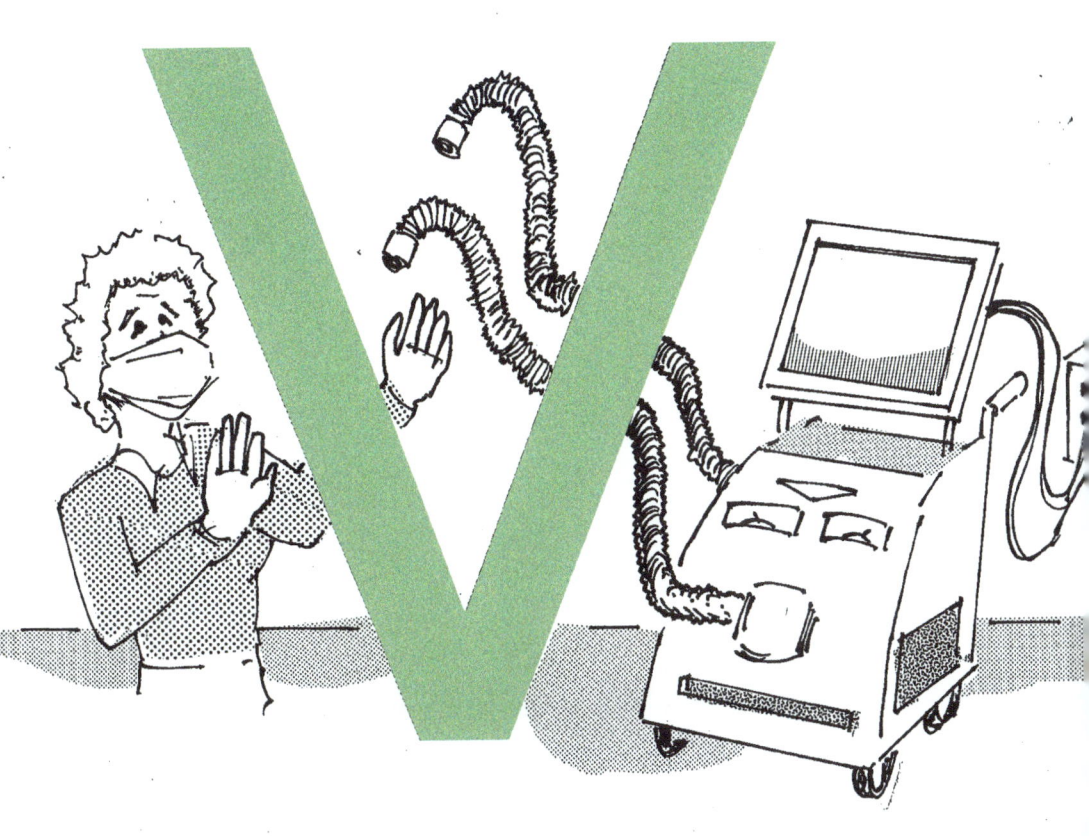

"When you arise in the morning, think of what a precious privilege it is to be alive –to breathe, to think, to enjoy, to love."

– MARCUS AURELIUS

"Be fast, have no regrets. If you need to be right before you move you will never win."

— **MIKE RYAN** 7NEWS.com.au 06/03/2021

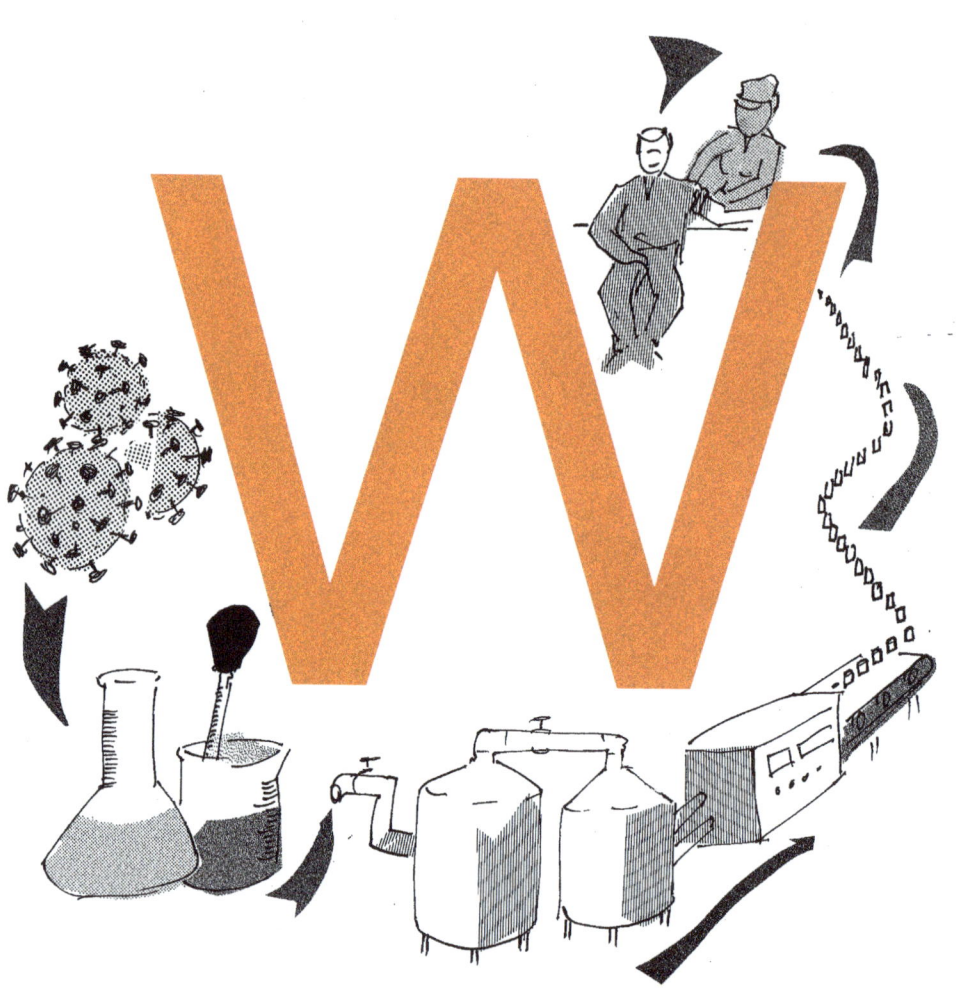

WARP SPEED VACCINES

Borrowed from science fiction, this term simply means, "at the fastest speed possible."

The Trump administration named the effort to develop and distribute vaccines and therapeutics quickly, "Operation Warp Speed."

The first vaccine shots were administered in December 2020. In order to reach herd immunity to COVID-19 a very large percentage of the population had to be vaccinated.

Sadly, the populations most devastated by the disease were not initially trusting of the vaccine. This was partially due to historic racism in medical research.

XENOPHOBIA

Fear, hatred, and attacks increased against those who were perceived to be foreigners blamed for bringing in the virus.

Because the virus originated in China, many people unfairly held Asian people of all nationalities responsible for the virus.

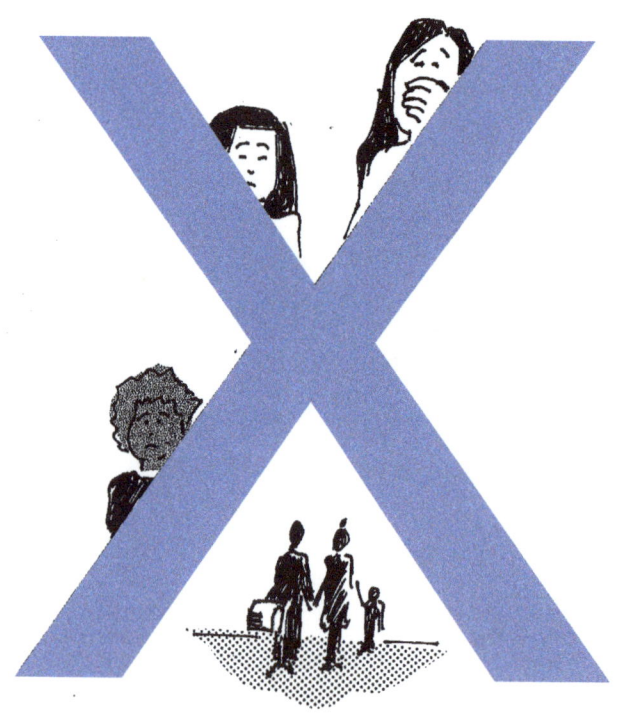

"If he were allowed contact with foreigners he would discover that they are creatures similar to himself and that most of what he has been told about them is lies."

– GEORGE ORWELL

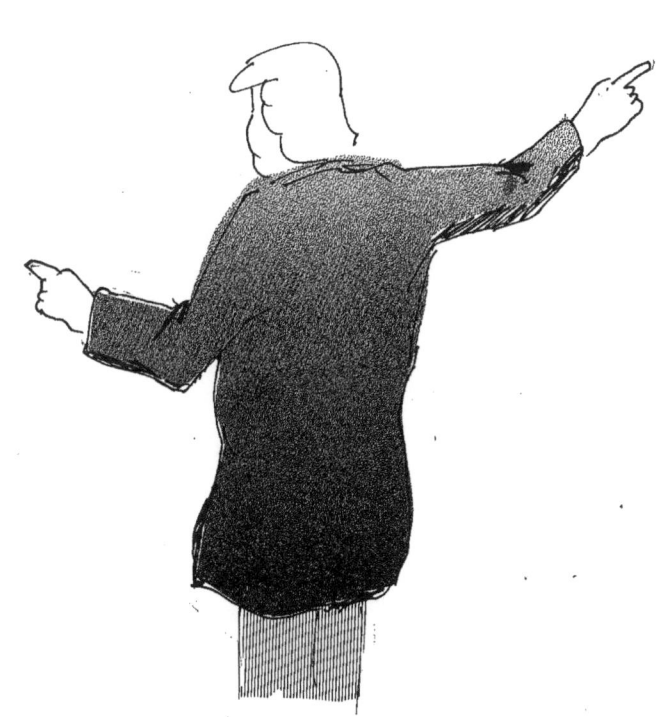

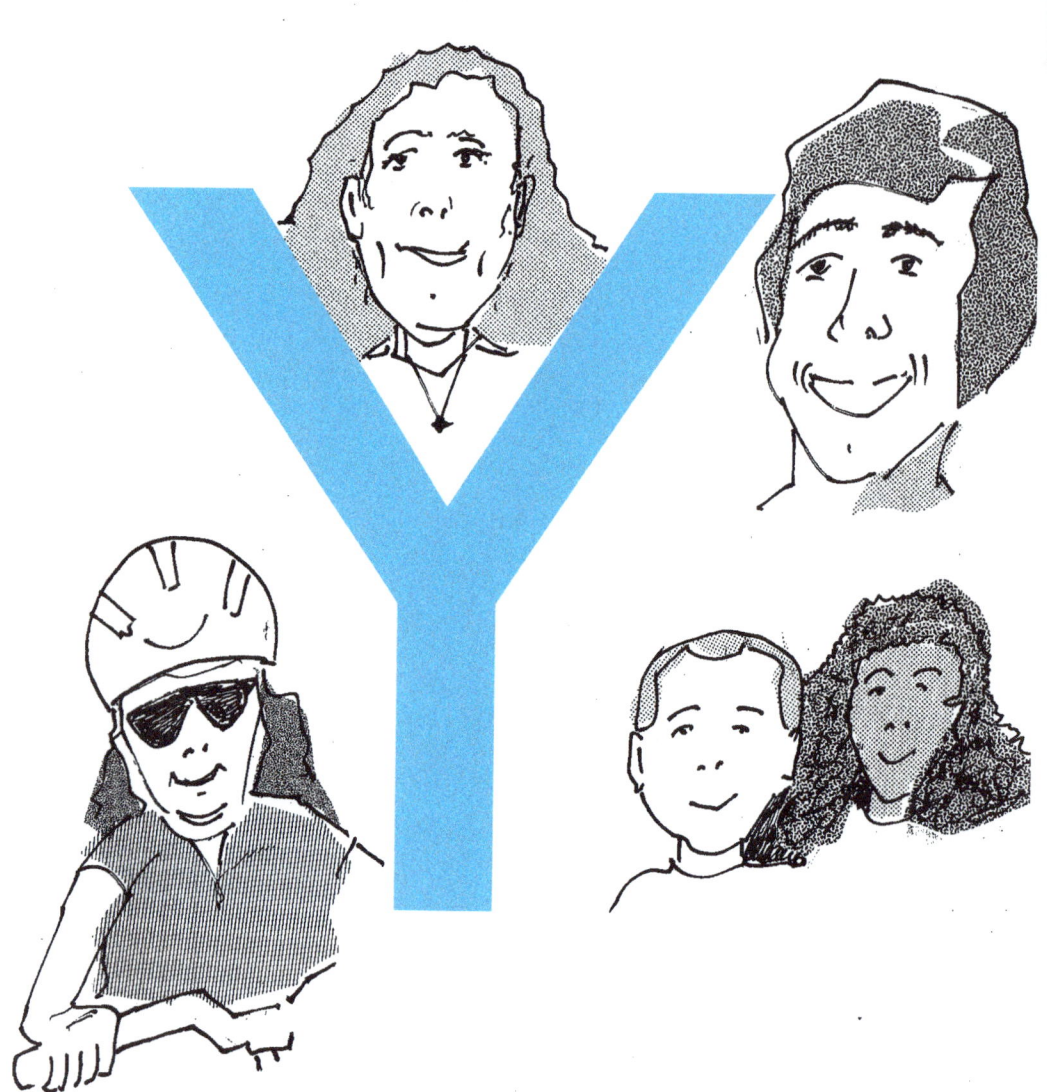

YOUTH

Early on, young people were thought to have been spared by the virus. In fact, COVID-19 was found to infect all ages.

Some children developed a serious multi-organ inflammatory condition.

Many of the 20-to-40 year-old cohort dared to challenge the virus at massive social gatherings known as "COVID parties," and jeopardized the lives of others.

"Facts do not cease to exist because they are ignored."
– ALDOUS HUXLEY

ZOOM

This video conferencing application was relatively unknown before the pandemic, but became a staple of social distancing.

Zoom replaced many in-person interactions like school, work, health consultations, family gatherings, parties, and cultural enrichment.

The "Zoom culture" gave rise to its own vocabulary, like "you're on mute," etiquette, and dress codes (concerned only with what was worn from the waist up).

Many people suffered from "Zoom fatigue," another manifestation of COVID isolation.

"Let us always meet each other with a smile."
—MOTHER TERESA

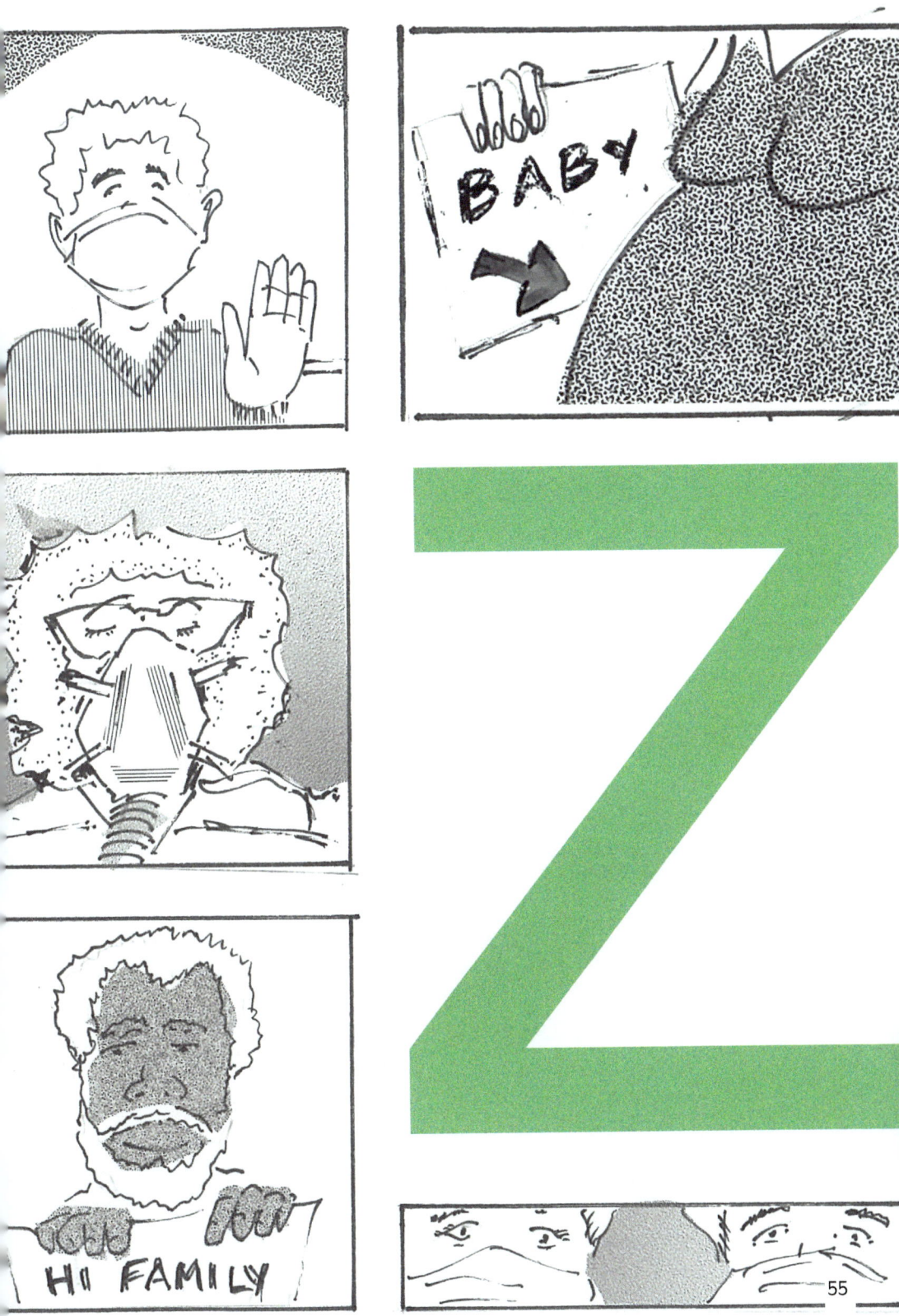

"Wow, thanks Pop, that was a good way to brainstorm. I have a lot of ideas now for more research," said Henry.

Thump, thump, thump, thump... "What's that?" Thomas asked. Pop looked puzzled. Mom and Mo were home from their shopping trip. To the guys' surprise the head of a neon Pterodactyl entered the room. Mo and Mom carried the back end. "Look what we found! Dino Drive-In is closing and discarding their props. This will be awesome hanging in your room," said Mom. Mo came over for hugs. The boys then stowed their stuff and changed out of their school clothes.

"Dinner is at 6:45, be sure you both are home on time. You can help Dad hang the dino after we eat," said Mom.

"OK," Henry agrees. "We're heading to the beach to meet Arthur and Leon. Leon just got his license and when Aunt Emily got her new all-electric car, she gave him her vintage CrossTrek. It's cool, Uncle Wayne souped it up. It's bright orange and it's a hot set of wheels for our boards.

See ya later -surf's up!"

AUTHORS

Emily Pogers lives with her husband in a Connecticut lake community. She enjoys reading alone, with grandkids, or with children in a nearby elementary school. She is retired from a career in medical product development; pharmaceuticals and instrumentation.

COVID-19 related "stay at home" orders eliminated her usual pursuits. Emily suggested using the time to connect virtually with family while learning self-publishing in a creative collaborative effort. Our result is "Viral Vocabulary."

A lifelong book lover, Maureen Pinney Casamassimo lives in Columbus Ohio. Raising three children and watching the growth of grandkids allows continued enjoyment of the written word. A career in clinical and school counseling reinforced the need for young people to hold a book, hear a book and unplug to experience real life, history and truth.

The opportunity to contribute to the development of "Viral Vocabulary" provided connection to create with family in a time when being together was denied. It will also serve as a family legacy for the generations to come. Maureen is married to Paul.

ILLUSTRATOR

Paul Casamassimo is a retired university professor, who specialized in making children smile. His life-long affection for doodling and caricatures led him to this family effort to describe humanity's response to the COVID-19 pandemic of 2020. Paul is Emily's brother.

DESIGNER

Dory is a designer that weathered COVID-19 with her husband and two children at their apartment in Queens, NY. She currently works for Uncle Sam, but is Paul and Maureen's niece. Emily is her mom.

www.ingramcontent.com/pod-product-compliance
Lightning Source LLC
Chambersburg PA
CBHW042048290426

44109CB00006B/153